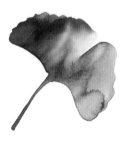

PURE SKIN

ピュアな肌

ピュアな肌

# PURE SKIN

## DISCOVER THE JAPANESE
## RITUAL OF GLOWING

*VICTORIA TSAI*

Clarkson Potter/Publishers
New York

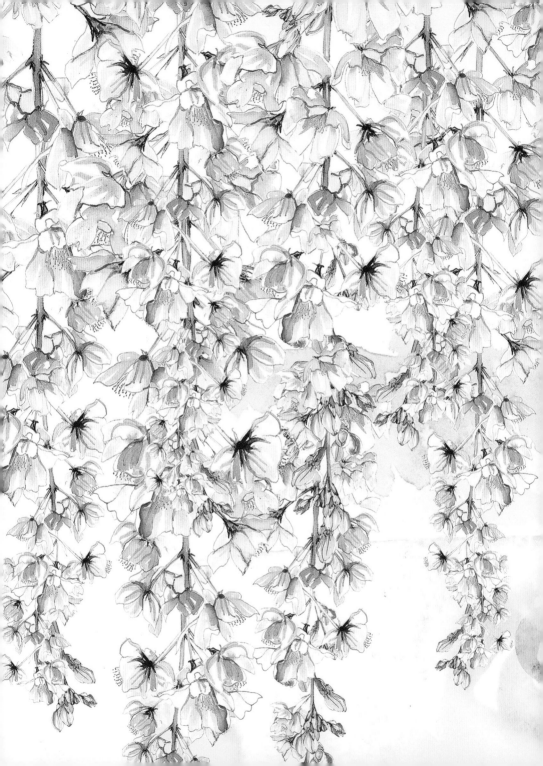

*This book is dedicated to the men and women of Kyoto whom I met along my journeys, for teaching me a different approach to beauty and life.*

*And to our Tatcha clients, for the honor of taking care of your skin.*

CONTENTS

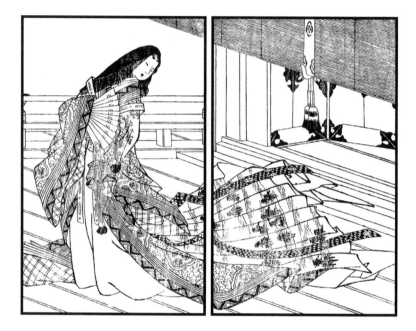

*Introduction: My Journey*

In the hustle of everyday life, do you ever look around and wish you could have a fresh start? I have.

My parents are from Taiwan, but I grew up in the United States and followed a Western skin care routine, like you may have. I always had good skin as a child and a teen, but when I did have an issue, I treated it aggressively. This was my approach for years, until one day it stopped working.

Seemingly overnight, I developed acute dermatitis. My entire face was covered with red, blistering, cracked, and scaling skin—not even my lips or eyelids were spared. I have always loved meeting new people, but during that time I withdrew from the world around me. I kept my head down and rarely smiled. I just wanted to hide. Desperate to reverse my skin condition, I tried everything: luxury creams, DIY serums, prescription oral and topical antibiotics and steroids—to no avail. It was disheartening to imagine that this skin was simply my new normal.

After graduate school, my work brought me to China twice a month, always with a short layover in Japan. On one of these trips, a friend in Tokyo introduced me to traditional blotting papers that absorbed my facial oil without irritating my inflamed skin. It was the first beauty product I could use without worry. In fact, the gentle sheets seemed to calm my complexion. Fascinated, I went to visit the artisans in Japan who made these beautiful gold-flecked, petal-like papers. I wanted to bring them to women in the United States, and asked how the artisans knew that the papers could be used to absorb oil. They told me that the geisha had been using them for centuries, and even offered to arrange a meeting so I could learn more for myself.

This was the start of an incredible journey that would forever change my approach to skin care, beauty, and life. During the summer of 2008, while pregnant with my daughter, I met my first geisha. I didn't know what to expect—in truth, I didn't even realize at the time that geisha still existed.

Suzuka, whose named translates to "cool fragrance," floated into the teahouse dressed in a kimono—the light purple exactly the color of wisteria—and wearing the iconic white makeup. She was so outwardly exquisite, so innately joyful, that I nearly cried. Her sublime beauty seemed to light up the room. It was a particularly warm afternoon, and Suzuka and I talked for hours. She told me all about her devotion to Japanese artistry, but mostly I recall that she didn't once perspire even though she wore a kimono. Only her graceful porcelain neck was exposed. Meanwhile, I knelt on my damp, slippery calves, sipped my green tea, and secretly prayed for a gentle breeze. My suspicion that geisha possessed special wisdom was confirmed when she smiled and said, "We don't sweat. It would not be elegant."

Suzuka taught me about the Japanese beauty ritual that geisha have loyally practiced for centuries. I learned that the classical Japanese approach to skin care is fundamentally different from what I had grown up with: instead of seeking to look perpetually twenty years old, geisha focus on having the best skin of their lives at any age.

After that visit, I asked my Japanese friend Yuko to help me research why these centuries-old gentle treatments and natural ingredients were still favored by geisha and modern women throughout Japan. She brought me to a traditional apothecary in Kyoto and taught me how to cleanse with camellia oil and mix rice powder with water to make an exfoliating treatment. I returned home with a bevy of mysterious products to try. You can imagine my surprise when, after three years with dermatitis, my face started to heal in just four weeks; after two months passed, my skin was fully restored.

Not only did this new approach to skin care give me my face back, but it also taught me a new way to consider beauty, and my own life. Each week, as my skin improved, I felt more order and balance. For me, adopting this Japanese skin care ritual allowed me to take back control and transcend the pace of the everyday. The experience of touching my face as I cleansed was a reminder to love and celebrate my skin, bringing a sense of calm to my soul. Now caring for my skin is a special moment and meditation, not a chore.

Inspired by my discovery of those delicate blotting papers, I launched my skin care brand, Tatcha, in 2009. The name was inspired by nature, specifically *tachibana*, the oldest, most formal practice of the Japanese art of flower designing. The name of this minimalist practice translates to "standing flower" and features only a few meticulously selected stems positioned in the center of a vessel. I chose this reference because it honors the Japanese appreciation for the beauty found in simplicity. As a Western woman and therefore an outsider to this world, I have been fortunate to learn so much about this unique and profound culture thanks to a team of geisha, researchers, and skin care scientists in Japan—all of whom have become my extended family. I feel like I have been granted permission to share a secret with the world.

I hope this book helps bring you to an awakening like the one I had. Within these pages, I will introduce you to geisha and the classical Japanese beauty rituals they embody. You will learn why their timeless four-step skin care ritual still comprises the core of every modern Japanese woman's beauty regimen. You will discover your own skin type, and I'll help you create a beauty ritual with ingredients tailored to your specific needs.

The lessons I have learned from the geisha and my new friends healed me in the truest sense of the word. What began as a search for skin care opened my eyes to a different approach to life and a discovery that your skin can be a reflection of your life's story.

Join me. Let's take this journey together.

# GEISHA
# BEAUTY

# MEET THE GEISHA

When people ask me to describe a geisha, I start with her title: *geisha* literally translates to "art person." These elusive women devote themselves entirely to classical art forms like dancing, playing instruments, arranging flowers, and brokering social diplomacy. (The idea that geisha are modern-day courtesans is a misconception born out of World War II.) Geisha culture is alive and well in a few cities, but I have spent my time mostly with those in Kyoto. In case you don't have the chance to meet a geisha in person, you may want to read one of my favorite books, *A Geisha's Journey: My Life as a Kyoto Apprentice*. This book describes the path to becoming a geisha as akin to the trajectory of a prima ballerina. A young woman starts training as early as fifteen years old, and after one year of intense daily tutelage in an *okiya*, or geisha house, she is tested before elevating to the rank of a *maiko*, an apprentice geisha, which is a title unique to trainees in Kyoto.

But that's just the beginning of her journey. Maiko then dedicate an average of three to five years to training and performing before they graduate to the status of an actual geisha, or *geiko* as they are known in Kyoto (while I refer to them as "geisha" in this book, the women I studied with were actually geiko from Kyoto). A geisha's typical working day starts in the morning with three hours of intense arts training followed by another six to eight hours of performances and appearances. Of course, that schedule doesn't account for her prep time to don an ornate ceremonial kimono with padded hems that can weigh more than thirty pounds. They are assisted by professional male dressers called *otokoshi*, the only men allowed in an okiya.

After dressing, geisha apply their classical makeup: opaque white foundation, defined brows, and crimson cupid-bow lips finished with

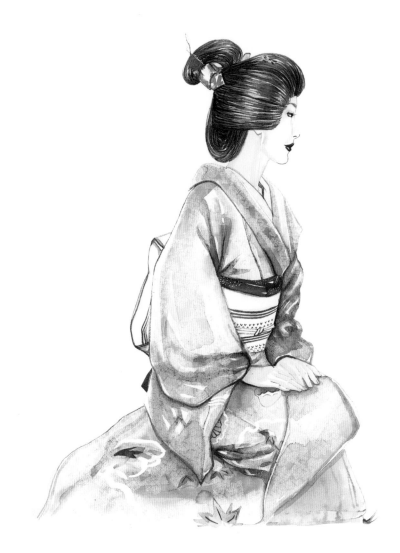

crystallized sugar as a gloss. Given the rigorous hours geisha keep, their physically demanding performances, and the full makeup they constantly wear, you wouldn't expect them to have beautiful complexions. But if you're ever lucky enough to spot a fresh-faced geisha of any age—from seventeen to seventy—you will marvel at her immaculate skin.

○まづ此のきざりを見るうちにて
見するやう

て
つる
べし
眉ざり
と上

○下のふとりをたんぞけ
下のことれふく
てたらべし

●下のふ
下のことれふく
てたらべし

○まごくの不目ふえざりやだんく
うとくまえろぐじまべてねいろて

△下のふとそれいろて
うもくぢりくく
おーろのときかえざら
やうまよえろぐじ

て天れぱし、洗ろれがさき立てんぐし

# THE JAPANESE BEAUTY BOOK

It's not hard to believe that geisha were once the "it girls" of Japanese society. For centuries, women sought to emulate their fashionable style, iconic makeup, and enchanting mannerisms. But unlike classic-era Hollywood movie stars who lived publicly and shared their beauty routines with their fans, these women were more ethereal beings who inhabited *karyukai*, or the Flower and Willow World. Their coveted beauty secrets were strictly passed along orally from generation to generation.

This tradition continued until 1813, when one enterprising author recorded the skin care and beauty fashions of the time in a three-volume tome known as the *Miyakofūzoku kewaiden* (Capital beauty and style handbook). My tireless cultural advisor and Tatcha colleague Nami unearthed an early copy of this treasure during our initial research of geisha beauty and wellness rituals. This timeless text is thought to be the oldest beauty book written in Japan and was reprinted for decades, but today, modern Japanese beauty executives don't know about it. When I mention the book in meetings, they wonder aloud why they have not studied—or heard of—this text.

What's most remarkable about the painstakingly recorded prepa-rations and intricate illustrations is their modern relevance. In fact, I pore over our translation regularly, as the content inspires many of our formulations at Tatcha. The vast majority of the book's skin care and beauty advice has withstood the test of time. The few excep-tions are understandable: the white makeup base once worn by geisha originally contained lead, so now it's formulated with rice powder. One of the original exfoliants—a paste of nightingale droppings—is no longer popular, for obvious reasons. But the book sometimes reads like a current issue of *Vogue*. There are how-to drawings for mastering

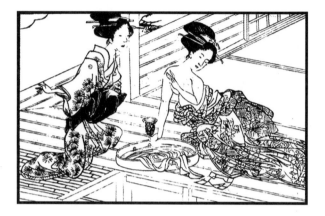

the perfect cat-eye and tips on how to contour your nose and shape your eyebrows. Even the centuries-old recorded skin care ingredients, from rice bran to camellia oil, are used today—and science has since proven their efficacy. Beginning on page 28, we'll explore these ingredients and formulate your personal beauty ritual.

○口の廣きなどでまく見るもの似
口の廣さへはよ日ふるとのから
美になのどく似ととあひ濃
ると付目に口益犬き渡きよ
人をつそりとてものどくまても
美おくく徐くく西うのし
口の廣きなのにろどくくれ
待くに推とろ唇の内へ物は
白都とおしりけてめるくくの
ゆく処日わどくろ唇の内
とろみくくとぶ被処と唇の内
とろみくどよみくく七ろ目わど

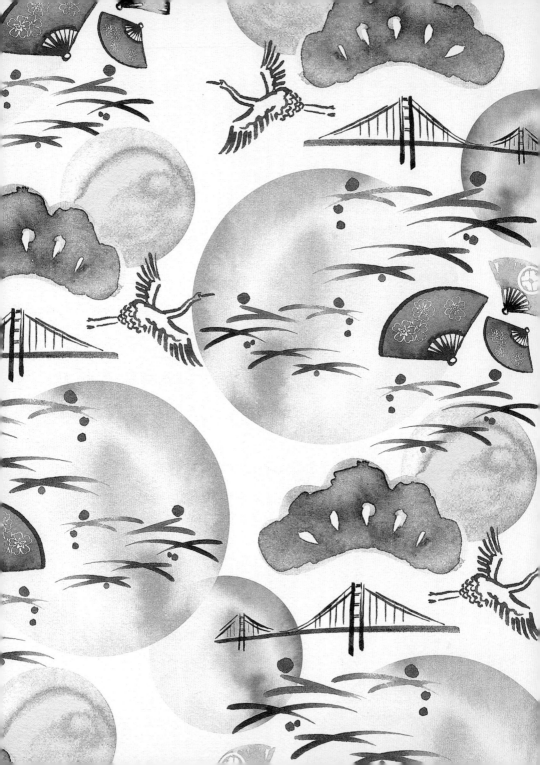

# EAST VERSUS WEST: WHAT I LEARNED ABOUT JAPANESE SKIN CARE

One of the first things I realized during my travels was that geisha and other Japanese women all have the remarkable, glowing skin we in the Western world associate with youth.

Before I embraced an Eastern-based beauty ritual, my relationship with my skin was often adversarial. I worked against it by using aggressive products that promised overnight transformation. When I talk to women with acne or eczema, they often tell me that they feel as if their skin has betrayed them. I understand that, because I thought of my skin as being out of control, too. But perhaps the most valuable lesson the Japanese approach to beauty has taught me is that skin care is about caring. Your skin works hard for you. If you show it attention and love, it will reward you with a healthy radiance.

There are a few other ways the Japanese approach differs from the Western approach, all of which we'll talk more about on the pages that follow.

**Less is more.**

Western women tend to focus much more on makeup than on skin care, accumulating an impressive collection of lipsticks, eye shadows, and highlighters from a young age. Japanese women instead prioritize a clear, smooth complexion using a curated skin care ritual. When it comes to both their arsenal of products and the ingredients within, they believe that less is more. Each cleanser, moisturizer, or treatment is a beloved and essential step, often formulated with the minimum number of ingredients to ensure efficacy.

**Ingredients are key.**

Japanese women are acutely aware of the fact that their skin is a reflection of their health. They know to avoid certain foods or to have a very plant-rich, clean diet for healthy skin. Many of the ingredients that are commonly found in their diet are also used in their skin care; it stands to reason that what is healthy for the body is also healthy for the skin. The basics of the Japanese diet—rice, seaweed, and green tea—are beloved ingredients even in modern skin care formulas. The idea of diet-skin connection is still a nascent concept in the Western world.

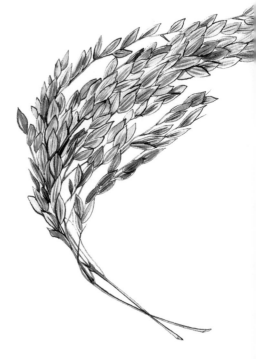

**Rituals are essential.**

To honor a ritual is to elevate an everyday action into something mindful, even healing. A geisha's skin care routine is necessary to melt away her makeup and keep her complexion clear, but it is not a daily chore. Whether it is the first time or the hundredth, the act of purifying the skin and massaging on a moisturizer is performed with precision and care.

**Skin care is self-care.**

The Japanese skin care ritual isn't about overnight transformations or aggressive treatments. Rather, it's about meditative moments of attending to your skin and therefore to yourself, every single day. To truly care for your skin, you must go beyond eliminating a pimple or splashing away makeup. Think of your skin as a reflection of your body. Could it be stress that causes a breakout? A lack of sleep that results in dry or dull skin? Lotions and potions will only go so far if you aren't paying attention to the state of your soul.

# THE
# GEISHA
# RITUAL

When I first began meeting with geisha, they would schedule our interviews in between their formal appointments. I only saw them in their flowing silk kimonos with delicately painted white faces and bright vermilion lips. Photographs rarely do justice to their otherworldly appearance because the camera flash bounces off the opaque white foundation and creates a harsh effect in photography. In person, the geisha's makeup actually glows under the moonlight and has an almost transparent quality.

As the geisha began to welcome me into their private world, I started to spend time with them as they rested in between classes— sometimes without their ceremonial makeup. When I saw a fresh-faced geisha for the very first time, I was absolutely transfixed by her natural radiance. Beneath the *oshiroi*, or white base, she usually wore was the most breathtakingly pure skin I had ever seen. After meeting many maiko and geiko of all ages over the years, I now know that this geisha was not an anomaly. The Japanese actually have a name for this supple, luminous complexion. They call it *mochi hada*, or "rice-cake skin," which refers to the flawless quality of a baby's skin.

I had to find out how they obtained and maintained such envious complexions. My immediate assumption was that their skin care regimen was as arduous as their arts training. I suspected that they devoted a great deal of time, effort, and money to it. Okasan, a former geisha who went on to establish a leading training house for geisha, taught me that their beauty ritual is based on classical Japanese principles and common ingredients. It's simple and straightforward. Even more compelling, the foundation for healthy skin is easy to master. You can tailor the ritual to your specific skin care needs. I'll show you how beginning on page 59, but first, let's look at the four steps.

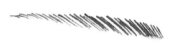

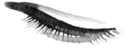
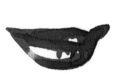

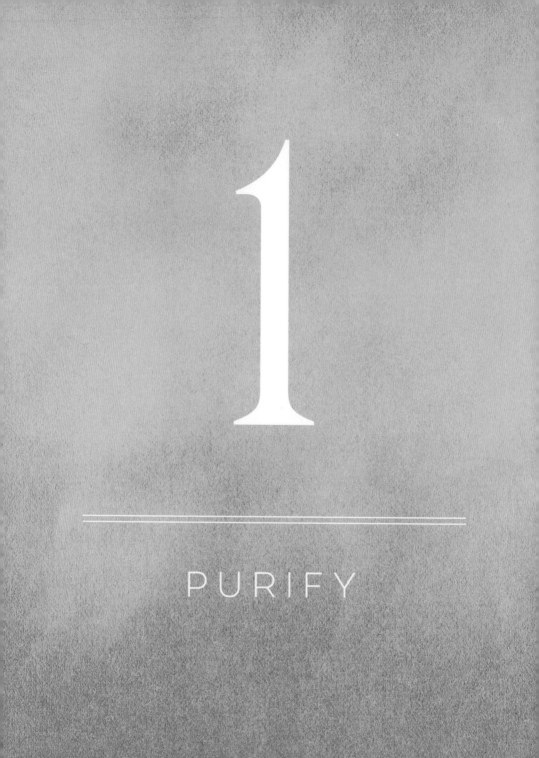

# 1

## PURIFY

Though cleansing is emphasized as key to healthy skin in Japan, that essential step is not a priority in the Western world. We tend to invest the majority of our beauty budget on moisturizers and serums while failing to wash away impurities like dirt, sweat, oil, sunscreen, and makeup. Choosing a cleanser is often an afterthought. The most important lesson I have learned from geisha is that cleansing is key to a clear, radiant complexion.

## Heritage

If anyone deeply understands the importance of gently removing cosmetics and debris at the end of a long evening, it is a young geisha or maiko. Imagine her makeup: after painting the opaque white foundation onto her face and neck, she also brushes on white powder and blush before she traces her brows, lines her eyes, and lacquers her lips in vivid red.

You might be shaking your head right now and saying, "But I don't wear that much makeup." Actually, we all do, if you consider the color cosmetics we use, like concealer, foundation, and highlighter or contour cream. The only difference is that we strive to look natural when we are made up, whereas geisha aim for otherworldly.

## Secret ingredient

You can imagine my surprise when I first learned that geisha cleanse away their makeup with camellia oil, the very same cooking oil used for creating marinades and sautéing tempura. Derived from a wildflower that flourishes in Japanese forests and is often called the "rose of winter," this petal-light oil is rich in oleic acid, along with vitamins A, B, D, and E. Camellia oil is also beloved in Japan as a leave-in conditioning hair treatment that seals in moisture.

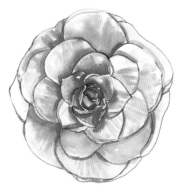

## Why it's essential

Washing your face with oil sounds counterintuitive, especially if your skin, like mine, veers toward shiny both in the morning and at the day's end. But water-based products and foaming cleansers can't solubilize or break down the natural sebum our skin produces—*or* the oils found in your makeup, particularly waterproof mascara and eyeliner. Like dissolves like, which is why oil works. So even your best soapy scrubbing effort at the sink won't remove makeup residue and stubborn sunscreen if you're not cleansing with oil.

Additionally, the harsh detergents in oil-free cleansers can strip away natural oils, and our skin reacts, sometimes panics, in response. Camellia oil contains anti-inflammatory, skin-softening omega-3 fatty acids that promote the barrier function of your skin. Macadamia nut and rice bran oils also make skin-loving cleansers, rich in essential vitamins and antioxidants without being comedogenic or blocking pores. If you have oily skin or an oily T-zone area, your skin produces extra sebum that can lead to clogged pores and eventually to breakouts. For a dry or sensitive complexion, this aggressive depletion of oil can cause rashes, tightness, and even fine lines due to dehydration.

## When it's most effective

In Japan, it is customary to cleanse the face twice a day, and I follow that lead. I purify as soon as I rise in the morning. You may choose to skip the cleansing oil step in the morning, since its primary function is to remove makeup, but I love the sensorial, spa-like experience of treating my skin. Think of this first foray into your classical beauty ritual as a meditative moment of self-care that sets you in balance for the day ahead.

Instead of waiting until bedtime to perform my end-of-day ritual, I cleanse my face with camellia oil in the evening right after I arrive home from work. In doing so, I envision that I am shedding any distractions or professional preoccupations that will interfere with precious time with my family.

**How to indulge**

To use cleansing oil, always begin with dry hands and a dry face. Fill your palm with a shallow well of oil and, using your fingertips, gently massage it onto your face—including around the eyes, plus lids—for 15 to 20 seconds. (Not all cleansing oils are safe for use around the eyes, so be sure to check the label.) Splash water onto your face and watch the oil quickly emulsify into a milky layer and effortlessly melt away makeup and debris. Rinse off with a few handfuls of warm water or softly wipe away with wet cotton pads. Oil cleansers are gentle and effective for all skin types. Just avoid cleansing oil formulas with mineral oil, which is known to clog pores, especially if you're prone to breakouts.

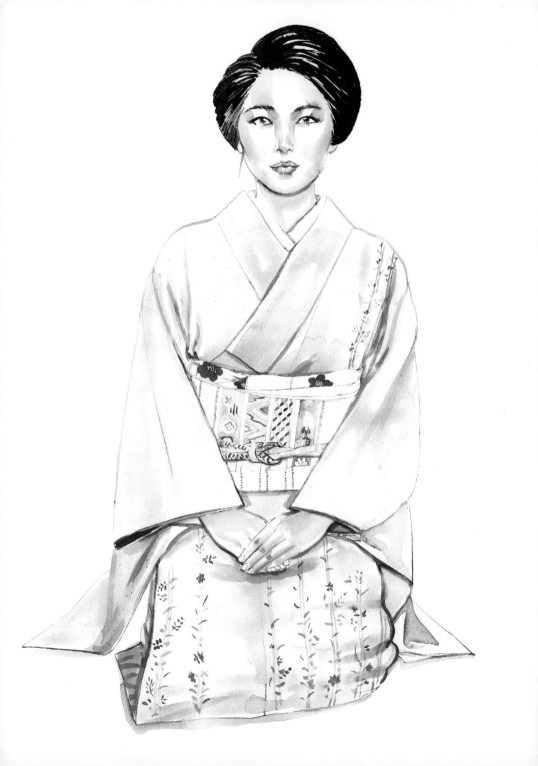

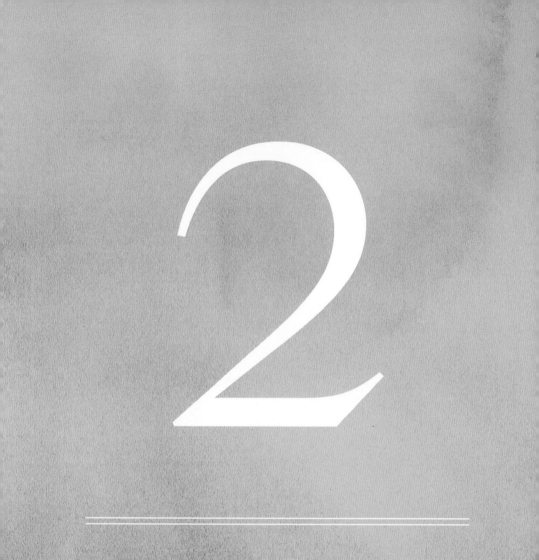

# 2

POLISH

Years ago, on a trip to Kyoto, I serendipitously discovered the classical skin polish that transformed the tone and texture of my skin. One afternoon, I visited a small boutique in the quaint neighborhood of Gion that geisha frequent for its snow-white face powder, ebony eyeliner, and other beauty items. Immediately, I was struck by how straightforward everything seemed in the tiny, softly lit jewel of a shop—especially compared to the sprawling, overstacked, and often confusing cosmetics counters in Western department stores.

As I browsed the narrow aisles, geisha came in and shopped with purpose. They knew exactly what they needed, and I watched many of them pick up strawberry-sized pouches of powder, tucked between rows of lacquer-handled lip brushes and sleek pots of pigment. I had to know more about these dainty satchels. A geisha explained to me that they were filled with finely milled rice powder for exfoliating the skin. Intrigued, I bought a few.

That night, once I rinsed away the powder, I was amazed by my skin's glow and newborn-like feel. In that moment, I realized that the luminous visage I sought with makeup, prescription topical ointments, and other treatments could be achieved with a commonplace and often overlooked ingredient like rice.

## Heritage

Before geisha apply their signature white base—which can highlight, rather than conceal, any skin imperfections—they must create the perfect canvas by pressing a light layer of wax known as *bintsuke-abura* onto their skin. This veil conceals pores, refines texture, and locks in moisture. (In essence, geisha have used face primer since hundreds of years ago.) To remove the wax and surface pollutants that collect on their skin throughout the day, they gently exfoliate their faces, often with this fine rice powder.

## Secret ingredient

Rice bran or *komenuka* has been a staple of Japanese beauty rituals for centuries because it's a vital source of vitamins A, $B_2$, $B_{12}$, and E, as well as naturally moisturizing proteins. Women used the leftover water from rinsing rice in their baths for soft, smooth, and luminous skin. In learning about this technique, I was reminded that my own mother and grandmother did this in Taiwan. They taught me to save this milky liquid known to soften my hands and add silkiness to my hair. Historically in Japan, grains were also ground down to make a gentle enzyme for the face and body.

## Why it's essential

This humble dietary staple effectively removes impurities while providing skin-nourishing oils. A natural enzyme exfoliant, rice bran boasts potent antioxidants and nourishing moisturizers. When activated with water, rice powder not only decongests your pores but also brightens skin tone, diminishes hyperpigmentation, and enables skin to better absorb the ingredients in the next steps in your ritual. Many conventional Western exfoliants contain seeds, salt, or ground shells that can tear and tug at the skin—even weekly use can cause irritation. Rice powders are beloved because they can be used everyday without stripping or pulling at your skin. Instead, the foam delicately removes the dead skin cells that make your complexion appear dull.

## When it's most effective
—

Exfoliate as the first step of your ritual in the morning (if you choose not to cleanse) and as the second step, after purifying skin, in the evening. As I gently massage the creamy rice bran foam into my skin, I think of the meditative mantra "Begin again." Rinsing away impurities and tired skin cells feels like I'm creating a fresh

start to my day and a new beginning for my skin.

## How to indulge
—

Many exfoliants contain harsh abrasives and can only be used weekly. For your daily polish, look for a rice enzyme powder that is gentle enough to be used every day. Wet your palms and splash a handful of warm water onto your face. Pour approximately half a teaspoon of powder (the size of a small coin) into one hand and gently rub your palms together to create a creamy, luxuriant foam. Massage gently onto your face with your fingertips in circular motions for 10 to 20 seconds, avoiding your eyes. Rinse well and pat your skin dry with a soft face cloth.

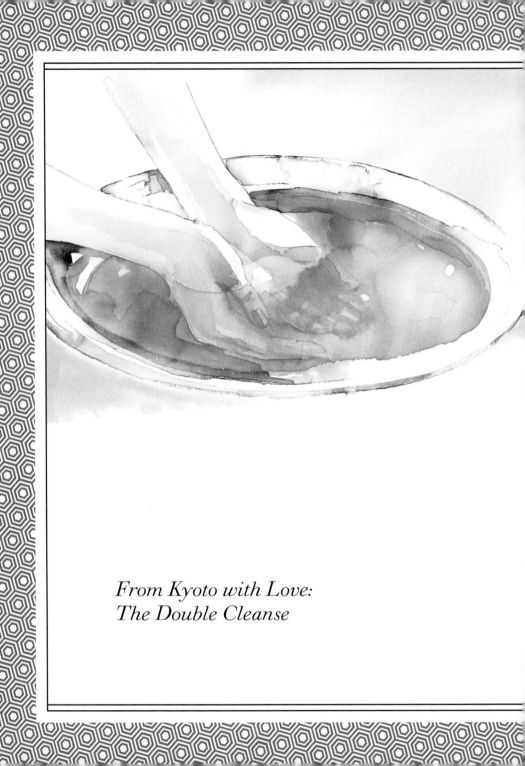

*From Kyoto with Love:*
*The Double Cleanse*

When it comes to purifying your face, myths and methods abound—and sometimes the beauty industry is complicit in re-inventing the playbook to sell you more products. You may have heard that a clean face should be as taut as a snare drum and squeak to the touch. Neither is true. In fact, your face should never feel tight; if it does, it's a sign that you have stripped away all of its natural and necessary oils.

The Kyoto Cleanse—also known as the Double Cleanse—is the two-step protocol favored by geisha and now throughout Japan, and it is already part of your ritual if you purify with oil and polish with enzyme powder. Those two steps not only remove surface debris, sunscreen, and makeup but also unclog pores and prep skin for hydration. In clinical studies, researchers have found that cleansing with oil and exfoliating with rice powder delivers results comparable to those one would typically expect only from an anti-aging moisturizer. The Kyoto Cleanse helps reduce the look of pore size; diminish the appearance of fine lines, wrinkles, and sun spots; and refine surface texture. Due to the popularity of Japanese beauty products, you should be able to find an oil cleanser and rice enzyme exfoliant easily. Lots of options are available.

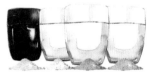

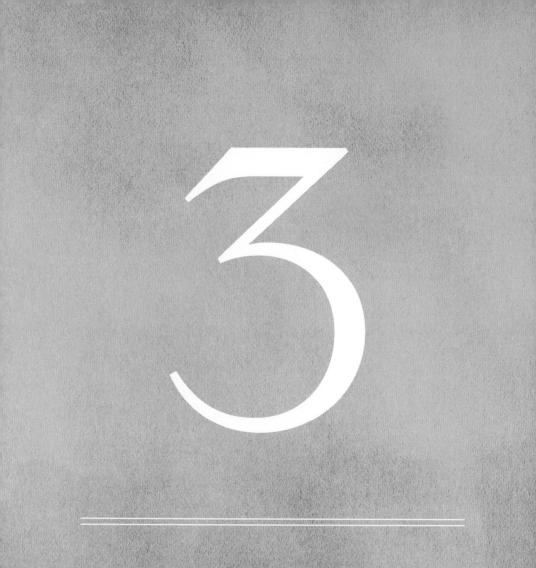

3

PLUMP

The Japanese skin care ritual has long been centered around "beauty waters." These botanical-infused essences, as thin and fragrance-free as fresh spring water, are a fundamental step in softening and brightening skin. When I first read about applying essence between cleansing and moisturizing, my skepticism was piqued. It seemed like an unnecessary and time-consuming detour from what could be a three-step ritual.

The fact that the majority of Japanese women today use an essence as part of their daily routine didn't convert me, either. In truth, I might have conflated essence with Western astringent, since they often look alike, and I may have still been traumatized from stripping my skin with alcohol-based toner throughout my teens. Rest assured, however, Eastern essence is very different.

Still unconvinced, I tried an essence that was in development in our lab in Tokyo; it was a pure fermented complex of green tea, seaweed, and rice. (To learn more about specific ingredients, see pages 81–95.) The morning after applying it, I awoke to plump, baby-soft skin.

## Heritage

Centuries before beauty waters were bottled, Japanese women harnessed the vital benefits of botanicals with an alchemical still or a system of tiered teakettles. This distillation technique was remarkably sophisticated for its time and involved boiling and steaming flowers to capture extracts in tiny cups to use as essence.

## Secret ingredients

The most efficacious essences rely on fermented nutrients that produce lactic acid, which aids in cell turnover and improves your skin's texture. Green tea, which is regarded as one of the most powerful antioxidants, targets free radicals, while seaweed contains natural polysaccharides, which replenish your skin's natural water reservoir and increase its capability to retain moisture.

## Why it's essential

Moisturizers must penetrate the skin in order to nurture. The top layer of your skin is made up of dead skin cells that protect the delicate skin beneath, but this layer can prevent active ingredients from sinking into the layers where they are most needed. A water-light essence floods skin with hydration and amplifies the performance of any treatment—including sheet masks (page 79) and serums—by channeling it into the skin.

## When it's most effective

The essence, which is patted onto the skin twice daily after polishing, should always precede any ritual enhancements like brightening serums, deep moisture treatments, or beauty oils. You may be so enamored with the plumpness of your skin and its resulting luster that you're tempted to skip the next step. Don't. The most important job of the essence and its primary function is to make the skin ready for whatever treatment follows. The essence is the first act of giving back to your skin after you have shed impurities by purifying and polishing. Though it takes only 7 seconds to apply essence, the act reminds me that many major life events happen in mere moments. Now that I am a devout believer in the plumping power of essence, I look forward to this part of my ritual the most.

## How to indulge

Use essence twice daily on a dry face, after cleansing and polishing—and before applying any additional skin care steps. Pour a shallow well of essence into one hand, press your palms together, and then gently press the essence onto the skin of your face, neck, and décolletage. Since the essence is nutrition for the skin, I look for products that do *not* list water as the first or a major ingredient. Avoid essences that note alcohol as a primary ingredient, because they will dry the skin. Also, cotton pads are for cleansing the skin with toners, not for plumping skin with essences. Don't waste this precious formula by letting half of it soak into a pad.

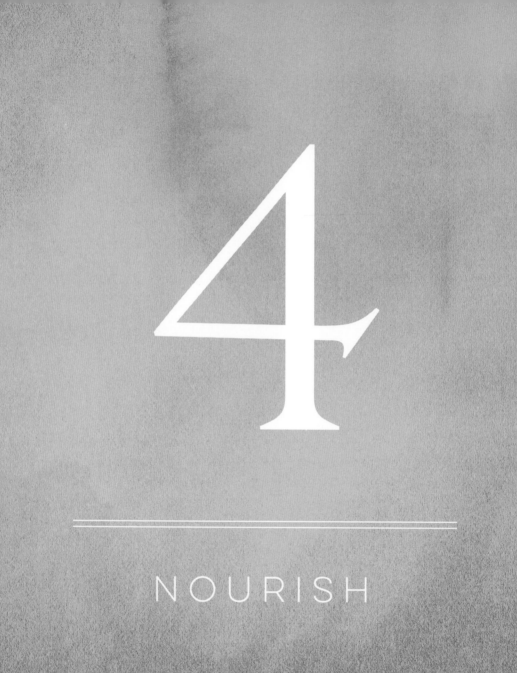

# 4

## NOURISH

I'll never forget my first visit to a workshop in Kyoto that specializes in silk and embroidery for custom kimonos. Inside, a Technicolor array of the sensuous, whisper-thin fabrics mesmerized me instantly. Thread shimmered on a loom and the sheen of finished fabrics swathed the room in opulence. When I pressed a delicate, cool-to-the-touch square of silk to my cheek, the natural fiber could have been mistaken for skin. It suddenly made sense to me why silk extract and silk protein are such popular ingredients in moisturizers, serums, and makeup.

## Heritage

Geisha saw the great value in silk for their skin early on. An illustration in the *Miyakofūzoku kewaiden* depicts young women poised over an elegant tub, washing themselves with swatches of the storied fabric. In Japan, silk workers have long been admired for their seemingly ageless hands—thanks to the protective layer created by the silky liquid in which their hands are often immersed.

## Secret ingredient

Silk has a protein- and amino acid–fortified structure that closely mirrors the composition of our skin. It's a miraculous material in that, much like our skin, it can keep you warm or cool as well as fluctuate its own pH. And silk can retain or repel water, just like our skin. It acts like a living material.

## Why it's essential

Silk extracts are easily absorbed into the skin, allowing powerful antioxidants and amino acids to help promote cell regeneration and condition the skin for improved elasticity and resilience.

## When it's most effective

Nourishment is always beneficial to your complexion, whether your skin tends to be more dry or oily. After plumping skin with an essence, apply moisturizer to form a protective barrier for your skin. When I nourish my skin in the morning and at night, I close my eyes and massage my face. It's a treasured moment of self-care that I never rush through. Sometimes, my daughter and I do it together.

### How to indulge

———

Use a small spoon to place a
pearl-sized amount of moisturizer, gel, or facial oil onto
your palm. Apply a dot to each
cheek, your chin, and your forehead. Then, using your fingertips, massage gently in upward
and outward strokes. My rule
for choosing a moisturizer is
to look for an antioxidant-rich
form that suits your skin type.
If your skin is dry, opt for a rich
cream or beauty oil. If your
skin is more oily in profile, try a
lighter gel or lotion.

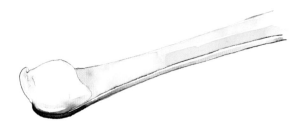

# A Silken Path to Softer Skin

There is an old saying in Kyoto: "If you look closely at a maiko's skin, it is made of pure silk." Even the *Miyakofūzoku kewaiden* references the luxurious natural fiber many times, and geisha relied on kimono scraps to wipe away their makeup. Long ago, treatises and precious documents were written out on silk paper, and a length of silk cloth was once so valuable that it was used as currency.

Here are five easy ways to pamper your skin with this precious material today.

## Eye mask

To cover your eyes when sleeping, reach for a silk eye mask. The long, nonabrasive fibers let skin breathe, unlike polyester or nylon. And with a smoother texture than cotton or linen, silk doesn't pull on the very delicate skin around the eyes.

## Sheets and pillowcases

Even as a fabric, silk has remarkable moisture-retaining properties, so your skin stays more hydrated during the night. Also, your mane glides across the slippery fabric, preventing the friction that can cause hair breakage.

## Scarf

Trying to prolong a blowout? Wrapping your hair in a silk scarf reduces its oil production and frizz.

### Skin care and makeup

You can find silk extracts, which are beautiful natural moisturizers, in products ranging from sheet masks to lipsticks. (See pages 46–47 to review protein-rich silk's myriad benefits for your complexion as a skin care ingredient.)

### Summer clothing

Hypoallergenic, cool to the touch, and breathable, silk makes an excellent and chic choice for hot-weather apparel. Always wear natural fibers in warmer months.

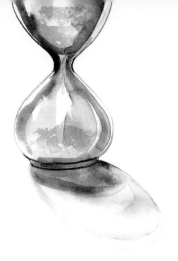

## SMALL MOMENTS FOR A BIG DIFFERENCE

It is a misconception that Asian skin care rituals have to be intensive, time-consuming regimens, often ten or eleven steps long. Quite the opposite, the classic rituals are as short and effortless as they are trans-formative for skin and soul alike. Giving yourself time to take care of your skin is not a luxury, but a necessity—a short, impactful moment for you to open and close the day. These few simple steps will translate into beauty for a lifetime. One to two minutes each morning and night will feel like a relaxing, mini-spa experience.

*Step One*

**Purify**

20 seconds to remove makeup and rinse or wipe away cleanser.

*Step Two*

**Polish**

20 seconds to create creamy foam in palms, apply in a circular motion evenly with fingertips, and rinse away.

*Step Three*

**Plump**

7 seconds to press essence onto dry skin and allow it to absorb.

*Step Four*

**Nourish**

20 seconds to apply cream or oil evenly in upward and outward strokes—if desired, add 30 seconds to gently massage the face and neck. (For specific morning and night facial massages, refer to page 97–101.)

CREATE

YOUR

RITUAL

# DEMYSTIFY YOUR SKIN

"Tell me about your skin." This is my favorite conversation starter. Working in my mother's beauty boutique as a teen, I quickly learned that our skin tells the stories of our lives. It might reveal the climate where you live, what you like to eat, or how many hours of sleep you got the night before. Isn't it amazing how telling the face can be? Even more miraculous is the fact that our skin is regenerative and can improve in tone and texture in just two weeks. Often, however, when I invite women to talk to me about their skin, they will lean in close and whisper, "I have bad skin."

It breaks my heart to hear that—it's unlikely that you would ever be so critical of your other vital organs, such as your brain or your heart. Skin is the body's largest organ, and it is so much more than what holds us together. It's our beautiful and natural armor, our most reliable communicator, and thanks to the wonder of sensory perception, it's an astounding source of pleasure. Think of the happiness that comes with a caress of your cheek or a needed embrace. When my daughter unexpectedly reaches for my hand, I'm flooded with joy at her gentle touch.

In Asia, women have a far more nuanced understanding of their skin for two reasons. First, beauty is defined by a woman's natural complexion more than her makeup. While in America we might start experimenting with eyeshadow and bright red lipsticks in our teens, girls in Japan focus on developing a trusted skin care ritual. The beauty ideal in Asia is very skin-centric.

Second, in Asia there is an emphasis on understanding skin care science. In the United States, cosmetic products are not regulated by the Food and Drug Administration (FDA) and, therefore, brands can't make scientific claims about changing the form and function of skin. As a result, they must rely on hyperbolized, flashy marketing adjectives like "revolutionary radiance complex" to describe a product's effect on the skin. I call this strategy "the veil of pretty words." But if you open a brochure for a serum or essence in Japan, you will see detailed diagrams of skin and explanations of how a formula treats the skin on a cellular level. Women in Asia also look as much to the past as to the future for skin care knowledge and solutions.

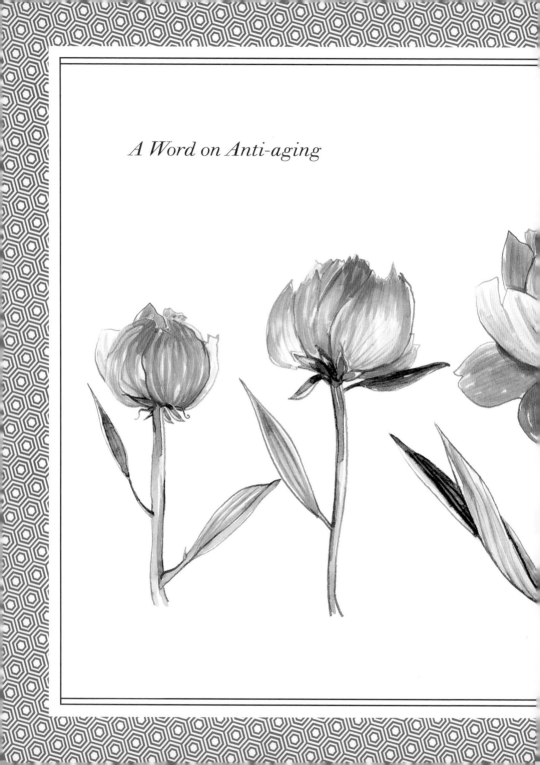

*A Word on Anti-aging*

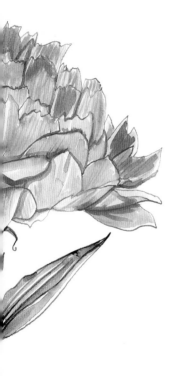

When considering your skin care routine, it's important to remember that our bodies were made to age. In Japan, aging is viewed as a gift rather than something to dread, as in Western countries. The goal is not to look perpetually twenty years old, which can result in "wind-tunnel face"—instead, the Japanese approach is about having the best skin of your life, at any age.

When I work with our team of skin care scientists, we formulate anti-aging skin care to minimize what is called "accelerated aging." This refers to anything outside your body's normal rate of aging and can be negatively impacted by a variety of conditions, including diet, stress, pollution, smoking, and, indeed, your skin care routine. If you've ever heard someone say, "Oh, she looks older than her years," they are referring to accelerated aging.

Maintaining a proper skin care ritual, along with a healthy lifestyle and diet, will help keep you as close as possible to the normal, biological rate of aging, rather than accelerating the process. Plus, it will minimize the look of aging.

# IDENTIFY YOUR SKIN TYPE

Knowledge is empowering, so caring for your skin begins with understanding its unique characteristics and needs. That way, you can adapt your ritual and choose options that create a healthier, more radiant complexion. Blotting papers—preferably ones made from abaca leaf, which won't dry out the face—make it easy to determine your skin profile in seconds.

First, gently pat (don't rub) a blotting paper on your nose, cheek, forehead, and chin before you wash your face in the morning. Second, hold the sheet up to the light to see how much oil is visible after you blot each area. If the sheet picked up little to no oil, you have dry skin. If the blotting sheet reveals some oil, perhaps taking up half the paper or less, your skin is normal/combination. Finally, if the blotting paper is saturated with oil and transparent, you have oily skin. Determining your skin type will help tailor your skin care to your needs, but the classical Japanese ritual works to make every type of complexion smooth, soft, and glowing.

A quick breakdown of the characteristics of your particular skin type follows.

# NORMAL/COMBINATION SKIN

**The good news:**

- Your skin is naturally balanced and happy. When it comes to a skin care ritual, less is more.

**You have normal skin if:**

- Your skin is comfortable throughout the day.
- You may get midday shine on your forehead, nose, and chin (the T-zone).
- Occasional breakouts occur, usually related to hormones or stress.

**Tips and tricks for normal skin:**

- Avoid aggressive treatments that can unsettle your happy balance.
- Your ideal moisturizer is a gel cream.

## OILY SKIN

——

**The good news:**

- Oily skin is youthful skin, which is cause to celebrate.

**You have oily skin if:**

- Your skin begins to shine shortly after washing it.
- You are prone to regular breakouts.

**Tips and tricks for oily skin:**

- Exfoliation and lightweight hydration are the keys to keeping your skin in balance.
- Your ideal moisturizer is a gel or lotion.

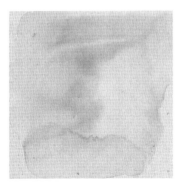

# DRY SKIN

---

**The good news:**

- Breakouts are behind you, and your skin laps up moisture.

**You have dry skin if:**

- Your skin yearns for hydration and occasionally feels tight.
- Breakouts are uncommon.
- You notice some fine lines and wrinkles.

**Tips and tricks for dry skin:**

- Dry skin loves pampering. Hydration enhancements and beauty oils will keep you glowing.
- Your ideal moisturizer is a rich cream or beauty oil.

———

**The good news:**

- Because you are diligent about using products and treatments that don't irritate your skin, your complexion is healthy. Your skin is communicating with you, and you already know how to treat it gently.

**You have sensitive skin if:**

- Your skin may be oily, dry, or normal, but it reacts to new products or environments.
- Eczema, dermatitis, and hives may occur regularly.

**Tips and tricks for sensitive skin:**

- Avoid synthetic fragrances and aggressive treatments.
- Your ideal moisturizer is fragrance-free and hypoallergenic.

**Sensitive skin can also be dry or oily.**

# A Lesson in Layers: How Your Skin Works

Once you have determined your skin's profile, it's helpful to understand how this spectacular organ works and which of its three layers most influence your complexion. Let's start at the bottom, where your skin is incredibly busy:

**The basal layer is the deepest layer of skin, where new cells constantly divide and nudge the older ones up to your epidermis, or top layer.** Hyperpigmentation starts down here where melanin is produced and acts as little umbrellas to protect your complexion from damaging UV rays. Sun exposure, hormonal fluctuations that cause melasma or patches of hyperpigmentation, and trauma to the skin (like acne) cause discoloration.

**The dermis or middle layer is where you find sweat glands, hair follicles, and the pockets that produce sebum or oil.** This level also brings blood to your face when you blush and flushes out toxins in the blood through vessels. Collagen and elastin are the main structural components of this layer, which give your skin volume.

**The epidermis is the outermost layer; it's what you see.** The epidermis regenerates regularly. Skin cells travel up from the basal layer to flake off about a month after they first form. Most of the things that we notice in our skin as we get older can be addressed through proper care of the epidermis, whether you are concerned about pore size, fine lines and wrinkles, discoloration, or breakouts.

This chart (below) shows the turnover rate of the epidermis's skin cells, which will drop as you age—it's why a skin care ritual is important at any time, but particularly impactful as we gain years (and wisdom).

**SKIN TURNOVER CYCLES**

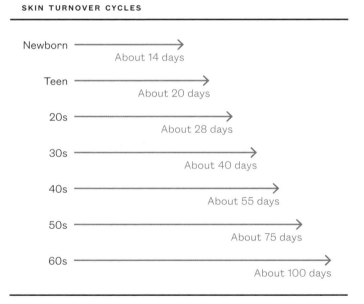

Newborn — About 14 days

Teen — About 20 days

20s — About 28 days

30s — About 40 days

40s — About 55 days

50s — About 75 days

60s — About 100 days

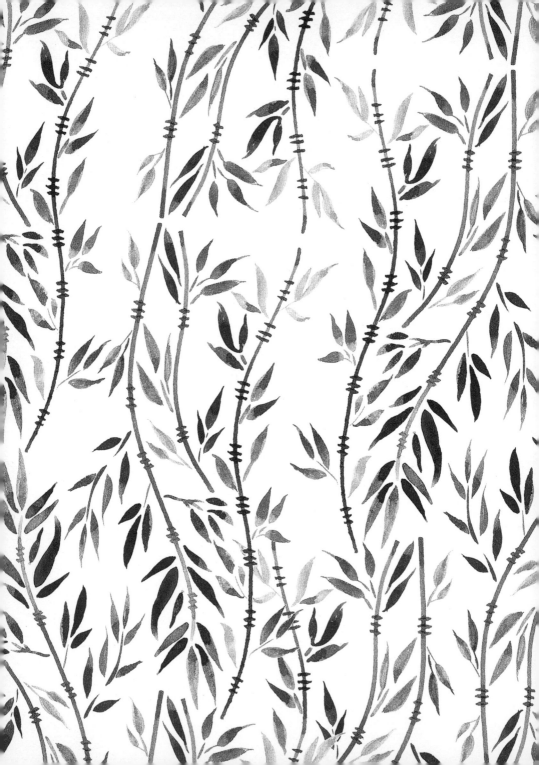

# WHAT'S YOUR SKIN CARE PSYCHE?

Beauty routines are personal and, in my opinion, an extension of your psyche—whether you're obsessed with the latest products or just thankful that facial wipes exist. Let's discover what your skin care type is, and look at how a new ritual might benefit you.

# You love to try the newest products and change up your beauty regimen frequently.

**Designing your ritual**

Although a life-changing formula may be just around the corner, your skin actually needs time to acclimate to new products. For example, it takes about two weeks to see the full results of a new moisturizer. The classical Japanese beauty ritual can be as simple or intricate as you'd like, while allowing your skin to improve on a realistic timeline. Give it time to take effect before moving on to new products.

# You have a tried-and-true regimen that has not changed for years.

———

**Designing your ritual**

It's wonderful that you have found products that work for you—no doubt the result of much searching. Do keep in mind that your skin naturally changes as you age, so your ritual may need to be updated to add hydration or reduce the appearance of fine lines and sun spots. A change of seasons or move to a new climate may call for a reevaluation as well. Because the four-step ritual can easily be enhanced with serums and sheet masks that work in tandem (see page 79), you can always recalibrate or enhance your usual routine—and see better results.

You address skin issues swiftly and assertively. You may have overexfoliated or overindulged with peels or other treatments in the past.

———

**Designing your ritual**

It can be so satisfying to focus on one skin issue until it's gone, but it would save you lots of effort to prevent the issue in the first place. By purifying, polishing, plumping, and nourishing your skin each and every day, you will help minimize those issues that drive you crazy, whether it's a breakout, dry texture, or sun spots. A classical Japanese ritual will help you prevent the issues, rather than address them after the fact.

Whether it's because you have a naturally compliment-worthy complexion or because you're too busy to indulge in your skin, you don't adhere to any particular beauty regimen, and you may not even wash your face every night.

—

**Designing your ritual**

There is nothing wrong with wanting to keep your routine streamlined and simple, but don't let the word *ritual* intimidate you. It can be completed in just a few steps, and in about a minute. All you need to do is purify, polish, plump, and nourish for your happiest, healthiest skin.

# ENHANCE YOUR RITUAL

# GET PERSONAL

The beauty of a classical Japanese skin care ritual lies in its simplicity. The four essential (and efficient) steps outlined on pages 28–51 cater to every skin type and any level of skin care enthusiast. Even once you've identified and created your best practices, factors like hormone levels, diet, travel, and weather can affect your complexion. You can tailor the basic ritual with enhancements that, based on your needs, will change from time to time, and over time.

| SKIN TYPE | ENHANCEMENTS |
|-----------|--------------|
| Normal | Facial mists are perfect for keeping your skin nourished and hydrated as needed throughout the day, but light enough to ensure that even oily patches won't be overloaded.<br><br>Blotting papers (look for all-natural, preferably abaca leaf) help lift away excess oil gently without stealing moisture from the skin. |
| Oily | Blotting papers (look for all-natural, 100 percent abaca leaf) help absorb excess oil from your face before it can clog your pores.<br><br>Brightening serum can help lighten acne scarring. |
| Dry | Hydrating sheet masks are perfect to replenish your skin's natural moisture reservoir.<br><br>Facial mists can hydrate and nourish skin with a quick spritz throughout the day. Avoid mists that are high in alcohol content; instead, look for mists that contain oils to help keep the moisture in. |
| Sensitive | Silk pillowcases are gentle and soothing on sensitive or compromised skin.<br><br>Colloidal oatmeal (in skin care or bathing soaps) helps calm skin irritations. |

# TIPS AND TRICKS FOR OPTIMUM SKIN CARE RESULTS

## CLEANSER

When using an oil cleanser or makeup remover, I like to do the "white towel test." Gently swipe a soft white towel on freshly cleansed face to ensure your makeup is fully removed. If not, it's time for a new product.

## EXFOLIANT

In the West, we often think of exfoliants as a weekly scrub, but using a gentle enzymatic exfoliant daily is key to cell turnover. If you feel any tightness or burning, your exfoliant is too strong. Instead, skin should feel pure, smooth, and soft.

## MOISTURIZER

Using fingertips or a soft brush, always apply in upward and outward strokes to counter gravity and dispel toxins from the face.

## EYE CREAM

With your fingertips, apply eye cream liberally in big circles around your eyes, down to the top of your cheekbones, and all the way up to your eyebrows. I think of the outline of Jackie O's huge, iconic sunglasses. Look for a rich texture with botanicals like peony and honeysuckle to nourish the skin.

## FACE MIST

Hold about six inches away and spritz one or two times all over your face. This can be done before applying makeup or after, for a natural glow. If your skin is dry again 10 minutes or fewer after applying the mist, there is too much alcohol in the formula. Avoid alcohol-laden formulas and instead look for the same nourishing and hydrating ingredients you would find in a face moisturizer, such as silk, olive-derived squalene, and hyaluronic acid.

___

### SERUM

Using your fingertips, massage serum into your skin in upward circular strokes. Because serums are known for their active ingredients, double-check formulas for safety. Avoid hydroquinone, which sensitizes the skin to the sun. If you're pregnant or nursing, avoid retinoids, which have been linked to birth defects. Instead, opt for licorice root extract, which is beloved for its ability to reduce the appearance of hyperpigmentation without sensitizing skin to the sun.

___

### BEAUTY OIL

Apply two or three drops to your fingertips and rub them together to warm the oil. Gently pat the oil all over your face, pressing it onto your skin. Choose oils that are noncomedogenic, like macadamia nut oil, rice bran oil, and camellia oil. Avoid mineral oil and other highly comedogenic oils like cocoa butter.

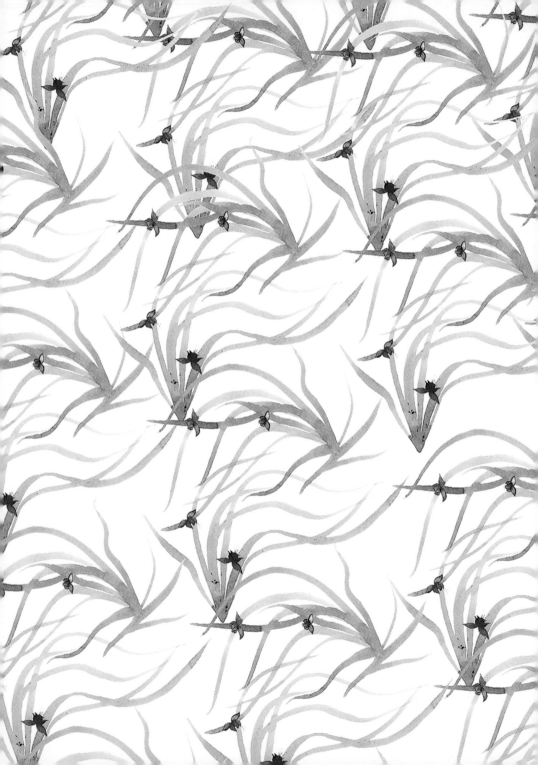

# SHEET MASKS DEMYSTIFIED

Sheet masks may be on-trend, but Japanese women have been indulging in this soothing, spa-like ritual regularly for centuries. I am often asked if these treatments actually work. They absolutely do.

A sheet mask offers the perfect opportunity to replenish the water reservoir of your skin. Drenched with serum or essence, the thin fabric or paper masks come in a sealed pouch and are immediately applied directly to a clean, makeup-free face for 15 to 20 minutes, then peeled off—the easy, no-mess application and removal make masks quick and convenient. The science is actually quite simple: the sheet material creates an occlusive layer like a second skin that prevents serum from evaporating, allowing it to fully penetrate your skin. Why is it so effective? A sheet mask doubles or triples the hydration of your skin—and you should not rinse your face after you remove it. That boost of hydration makes your complexion less vulnerable to free radicals that cause premature aging. Instead, seal that moisture into your skin by applying a beauty oil, lotion, or cream immediately after you remove the mask.

I set aside time on Sunday nights to give my skin a flood of hydration so it looks luminous heading into the week. I've made it part of my weekly ritual: I apply a mask and read a book to my daughter. And after a long flight, a sheet mask is the perfect way to restore hydration to your parched skin. (The humidity level on an airplane dips to half the level our skin needs to stay moisturized.) I usually apply a face mask as soon as I arrive at my hotel or as soon as I return home after a trip. Be sure to gently pat any extra serum or essence onto your neck, décolletage, and even the back of your hands before you discard the mask and packet.

# INGREDIENTS TO BELIEVE IN

I developed a keen awareness of how skin care ingredients affect our bodies when I was pregnant with my daughter. Skin is semipermeable, meaning things can pass through the skin and into our bodies—that's why treatments like nicotine patches are effective. With a baby growing, I felt prodded to review my arsenal of beauty products. My quest for a more thoughtful approach to skin care, in part, led me to the pure and holistic Eastern approach to beauty. In creating Tatcha, it was important to me to uphold a promise of pure ingredients free of formulations that can cause harm. Along with our skin care scientists in Japan, I examine the data on all the raw materials we use. We spend as much time on the materials as we do on the formulas themselves, and we keep working until we know the products are gentle, pure, and efficacious. While a formula doesn't have to be 100 percent natural to be good for you, natural ingredients can deliver impressive results without harmful side effects. Just like natural foods, natural ingredients give the body what it needs safely.

When I first shared with my team the ingredients recorded in the *Miyakofūzoku kewaiden*, they informed me that those ingredients have stood the test of time. Many botanicals and extracts that we know today to be beneficial to the skin or body were beloved in ancient medicine.

Let's look at seven traditional, pure Japanese ingredients that have been used for centuries, and tips on how to use them.

## History

The Japanese plum or loquat tree produces glossy green leaves that have been a popular medicinal treatment for at least three thousand years. During Japan's Nara period, between AD 710 and 794, the royal family founded a healthcare facility that relied heavily on this botanical.

## Why it works

Known as "healing fans," these tree leaves reduce skin inflammation when their extract is applied topically. The leaves also soothe edema and swelling from allergic reaction.

## Try it for

Calming sensitive skin and irritation from things like hives. Rich in vitamin C, loquat leaf extract also neutralizes free radicals that cause fine lines.

## Where to find it

Japanese moisturizers and topical creams.

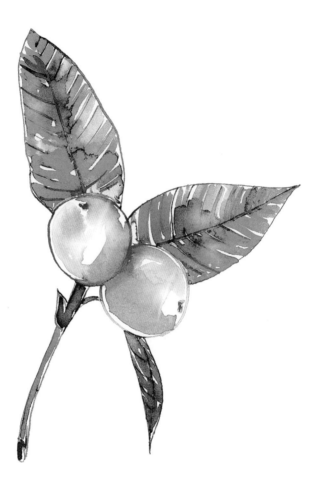

## History

For centuries, artisans in Kyoto have used this leaf to protect gold and other precious metals as they hammered them into delicate, thin sheets. They realized that the leaves left their hands feeling refreshed. Later, geisha and Kabuki actors began to use the leaves to set their makeup in place.

## Why it works

A relative of the banana tree, abaca is water-resistant and sturdy enough to be used in ropes on large ships, and yet gentle enough that artists craft woven fabrics from its pulp. This combination of strength and softness makes it perfect for lifting oil from the skin.

## Try it for

Setting makeup, like foundation and concealer. After application, blot away excess oil to keep makeup from looking heavy on the skin. You can also blot throughout the day to keep skin petal-fresh without disturbing makeup.

## Where to find it

Traditional Japanese blotting papers.

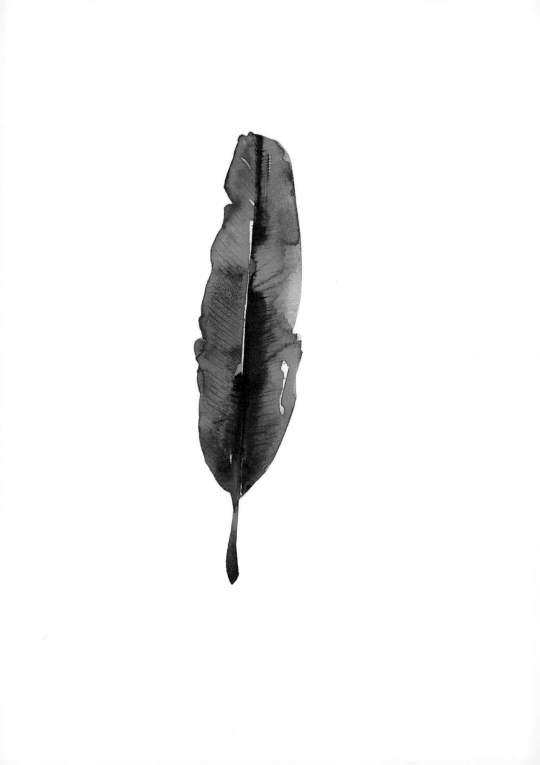

**History**

Women in Japan, who pride themselves on having porcelain skin even without makeup, recognized early on that the root extract of licorice brightens skin and evens out its tone. The extract was also known for rejuvenating energy and detoxifying the system in the case of poisoning.

**Why it works**

Licorice root is rich in glycyrrhizate, an agent that inhibits excess melanin production and helps to prevent hyperpigmentation. One extract, dipotassium glycyrrhizate, is a beloved anti-inflammatory and anti-irritant with skin-soothing properties. Another, glycyrrhetinic acid, has demonstrated anti-allergenic, antibacterial, and anti-inflammatory properties.

**Try it for**

Fading sun spots and preventing hyperpigmentation. Its skin-soothing properties also help calm rosacea and psoriasis.

**Where to find it**

Anti-aging serums, cleansers, masks, and moisturizers with skin-brightening benefits.

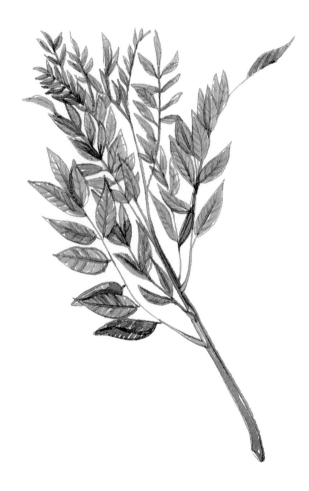

**History**

In traditional Eastern medicine, the leaves of this plant were used as a poultice to treat wounds. The rose hips became dietary supplements and herbal remedies for the flu, inflammation, and osteoarthritis. Water infused with dried rose petals was also served as a tea to relieve headaches.

**Why it works**

Abundant in vitamins A, C, and E, and rich in flavonoids and tannins, the fruits of this flower promote production of collagen and regulate the skin's natural barrier function.

**Try it for**

Minimizing the appearance of pores and boosting collagen synthesis to make skin more plump and firm.

**Where to find it**

Lip balms, body oils, and pore-perfecting products such as moisturizers, treatments for oily skin, and hydrating gels.

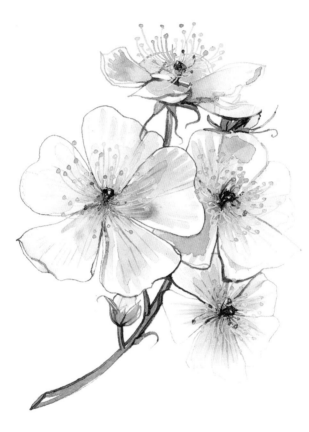

**History**

Historically, women have crushed pearls into powder to be taken medicinally—or to be mixed with water for a nourishing facial treatment. Centuries ago, royal families added pulverized pearl powder into their moisturizers and makeup for a luminous effect.

**Why it works**

Pearl acts as a potent antioxidant, boosting the body's own enzymes and reducing peroxidation or cell damage. Polysaccharides, amino acids, minerals, and proteins help replenish and rebuild skin.

**Try it for**

Firming skin, exfoliating dead cells, and brightening dark spots.

**Where to find it**

Exfoliants, sheet masks, and creams.

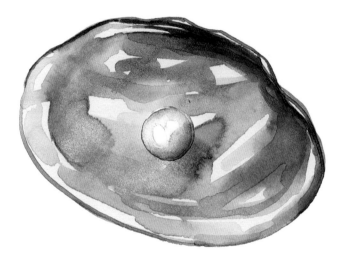

**History**

During the Edo period, samurai wore a layer of indigo-dyed cotton beneath their armor to help heal injuries. (In Japan, the color is often referred to as "samurai blue.") The rich dye was also used for traditional firefighter uniforms and presented to newborns in the form of an indigo-dyed blanket—a symbolic testament to its protective qualities.

**Why it works**

Indigo's active ingredients provide powerful anti-inflammatory relief. Tryptanthrin is a nitrogen-rich, antimicrobial compound that helps flush away toxins and irritants. Indirubin, a dynamic isometric compound, promotes the skin's healing abilities by strengthening its barrier function.

**Try it for**

Soothing symptoms of irritation from conditions like dermatitis, rosacea, psoriasis, and eczema.

**Where to find it**

Hand creams, beauty balms, body butter, and products formulated specifically for sensitive skin.

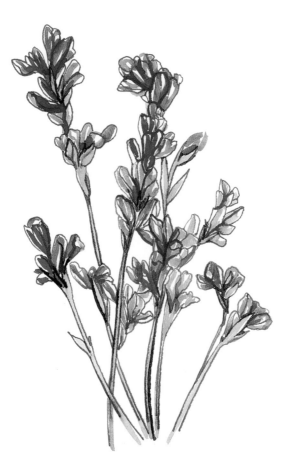

ALGAE

## History

Red algae is known on the Japanese island of Okinawa as "treasure from the god of the sea." For centuries, generations of fishermen have carefully harvested the algae from lagoons without disturbing the coral beneath. Also known as seaweed, algae has been incorporated into many beauty rituals for skin and hair alike. Red algae is so revered in Japan that it is presented as a temple offering during the traditional festivals of the Yaeyama district in Okinawa.

## Why it works

Red algae is rich in natural polysaccharides, the molecule that provides its incredible moisture-retaining properties. If you drop certain dried red algae in water, it instantly drinks up the moisture, blossoming and turning from a dull maroon into a vibrant red.

## Try it for

A burst of hydration for any skin type. Even oily skin can become dehydrated—red algae replenishes the skin's moisture reservoir for a plump, glowing complexion.

## Where to find it

Japanese moisturizers and hydrating face masks.

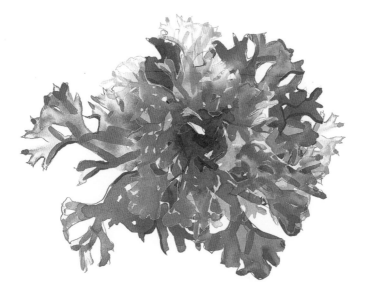

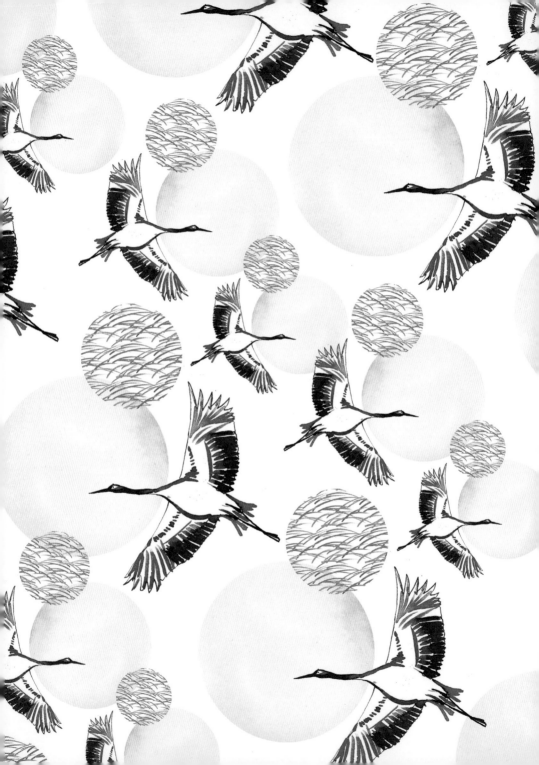

# FACIAL MASSAGE

Japanese facial massage may be one of my most cherished beauty regimen enhancements. This practice has been proven to de-puff your skin and promote microcirculation, which boosts blood flow to vessels that can build up with waste that causes dull skin and fine lines. This invigorating flow not only refreshes blood cells and removes that waste but also feels fantastic and adds just 2 minutes to your skin care ritual. Like me, you may be surprised by how quickly those precious moments pass.

I like to incorporate facial massages into both morning and evening rituals. In the morning, I massage my face with the purify step to stimulate my mind as well as my skin. In the evening, I perform a massage as I moisturize skin in the nourish step. There are many ways to perform facial massages, but the key is to always move upward and outward, from the center of the face.

*Asayake* means "morning glow" in Japanese. This type of massage calls for the palms to be chilled with cold water to tighten and awaken the skin. Repeat the following five-step process five times.

*Step One*     Apply moisturizer onto your hands to allow them to glide on the skin. (Refer back to pages 59–63 for the best moisturizer for your skin type.)

*Step Two*     Gently massage your hands up along your neck.

*Step Three*   Move upward from the center of your chin along the jawbone, applying light pressure.

*Step Four*    Lay your fingers against your nose and move outward along the orbital bone.

*Step Five*    Place your fingers above your eyebrows and glide upward toward the hairline.

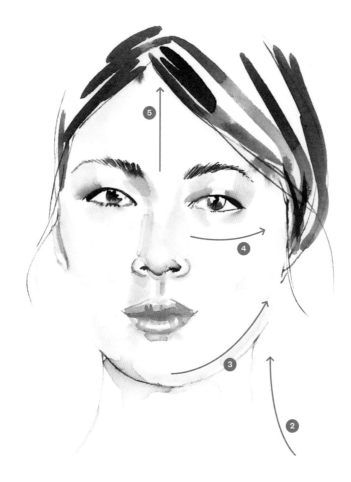

For this "evening glow" massage, which releases tension and detoxifies through lymphatic drainage, first rub your hands together to warm them. Then repeat the following four-step process five times.

*Step One*    Begin with your fingers just above the hairline and move away from the forehead in a back-and-forth motion on the scalp.

*Step Two*    Apply moisturizer onto your hands. Press your fingers above the inner corner of the eyebrows and slide outward along the brow, stopping in front of the ears.

*Step Three*    Press your forefingers and middle fingers at the base of the nose and move outward along cheekbones.

*Step Four*    Place your fingers behind your ears and draw down along the jaw and neck to the collarbone. This is the only downward motion you'll use, to encourage lymphatic drainage.

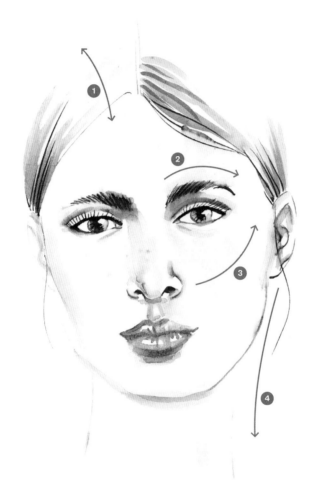

*RITUAL RESULTS*

# IMMEDIATELY,
## YOU SHOULD SEE . . .

- Increased hydration, with essence and moisturizers.
- Firmer skin, with sheet masks.
- Improved skin texture, with exfoliators.

# WITHIN TWO WEEKS,
## YOU SHOULD SEE . . .

- Improvement in fine lines and wrinkles, with moisturizers.
- Acne beginning to clear up, with exfoliatiors.
- Pore sizes beginning to diminish, with exfoliatiors.

# WITHIN ONE MONTH,
## YOU SHOULD SEE . . .

- Improvement in age spots and hyperpigmentation, with a daily brightening serum, daily exfoliating, and daily sun protection.

*Remember, while we are always looking for results when it comes to skin care, the true ethos of the classical Japanese skin care ritual is prevention. It's not just about the results that you see but the issues that you never see, if you take care of yourself a little bit every day.*

# BEYOND THE RITUAL

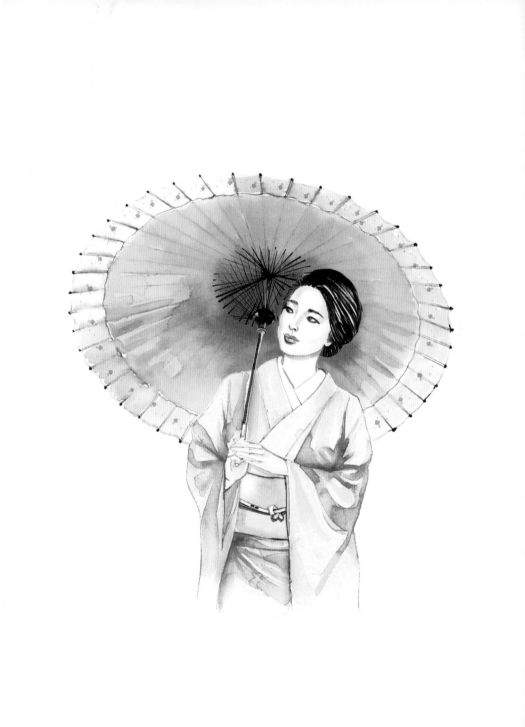

# SUNSCREEN IS NOT OPTIONAL

When I first started poring over geisha beauty rituals, I could find no record of sun protection other than the vibrant parasols they carry and twirl. How could they maintain their porcelain complexions without using some form of sunscreen, I wondered. The answer is in the oshiroi—or their snow-white foundation that contains zinc oxide, a mineral that sits on top of the skin and forms a barrier against the sun's harmful rays.

Modern Japanese women certainly don't wear oshiroi, but they are diligent in protecting their skin, even as teens. Many of them carry *higasa* or vivid parasols. They also cover nearly every exposed inch of skin by wearing big hats and visors, fingerless gloves, huge sunglasses, and even leggings beneath a skirt.

It may not be practical for you to be *so* fastidious in protecting yourself against the sun, but at the very least, you should wear sunscreen any time you go outside. In my opinion, learning about sunscreen should be as quick and easy as applying it. Let's go over what you need to know.

There are two types of sun rays: ultraviolet-A (UVA), which causes aging, and ultraviolet-B (UVB), which causes burning. UVA is sneaky and causes accelerated aging that you see in sun spots, while UVB is the culprit behind sunburns. Look for mineral-based sunscreens that contain zinc oxide or titanium dioxide and offer broad-spectrum coverage. That way, you're protected against both types of rays.

Levels of sun protection factor (SPF) that exceed 30 are not essential. An SPF of 30 deflects 96.7 percent of rays; an SPF of 50 protects against 98 percent. It is scientifically impossible to block 100 percent of rays. In fact, the FDA recently banned skin care companies from making claims over SPF 50 because that's as high as an SPF can effectively go.

——

Always apply sunscreen generously and cover your face, neck, ears, lips, and hands. (I use half a tube of sunscreen on my daughter, Alea, for a day at the beach.) Ultraviolet (UV) protective clothes and over-sized sunglasses make perfect summer-safe accessories.

# WHOLE-BODY BEAUTY

Too often, we focus on the face and ne-
glect the all-important skin on the rest of
our bodies. In Japan, however, beauty and
grooming routines are head-to-toe. The
Japanese shower before they enter the tub
to bathe, then soak to relax their muscles,
detox their bodies, and rejuvenate their
minds. The cultural emphasis is on carving
out a meditative moment of serenity and
calm in a fast-paced day.

*Onsen* translates to "hot springs,"
but the definition has come to include
the many spas that have soaking tubs fed
with mineral-rich waters from the jag-
ged volcanic areas of the country. A hot
spring law, called *onsenhou*, ensures that spa
proprietors don't use tap water or dilute the
mineral composition of spring waters. Even
a group of macaque monkeys, known as
snow monkeys, have their own onsen park
in a snowy forest in northern Japan. These
sweet and furry pink-faced primates sit
and soak with blissful smiles. Onsen are so
beloved that many Japanese homes include
a large, deep bathtub—often big enough
for two—with a view.

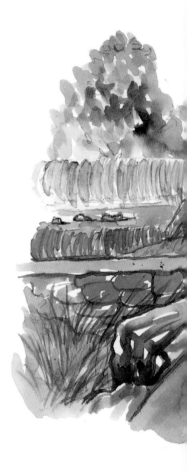

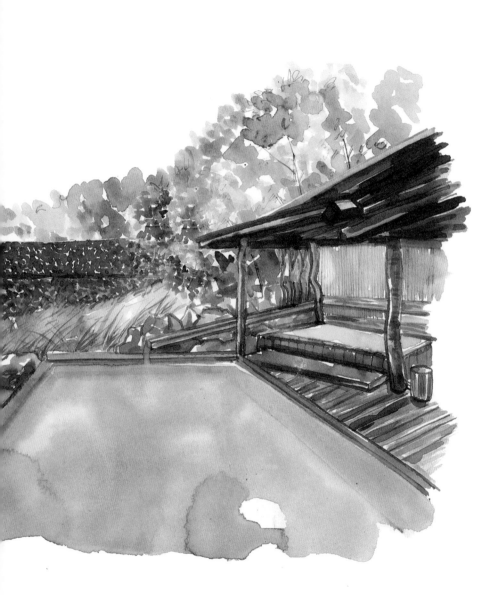

For your own onsen-inspired bath . . .

*Step One*    Shower first so the bath is just a time to relax and soak. The traditional first step of the practice is to buff the body with a silk washcloth in the shower. That way, you are already thoroughly cleansed, and your skin is prepped upon stepping into the tub.

*Step Two*    Traditional onsen bathwater is an aromatic cloud of tranquility, naturally enriched with sodium bicarbonate and sodium sulfate powders. Add a little something extra to the water, either for a fragrant effect or for benefits to the skin. In Japan, a citrus fruit called yuzu and other seasonal herbs are added. Try halved lemons or limes for a more refreshing soak. A splash of camellia oil will nourish and soften your skin. Hang dried eucalyptus branches in the bathroom to add an invigorating scent.

*Step Three*    Use a moisturizer immediately after you soak—or even after you take a reflective shower—to seal in the hydration. Pat or blot your skin with a towel until you are just barely dry before applying the moisturizer.

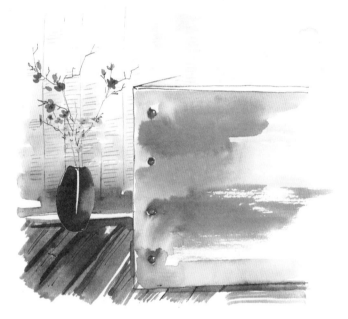

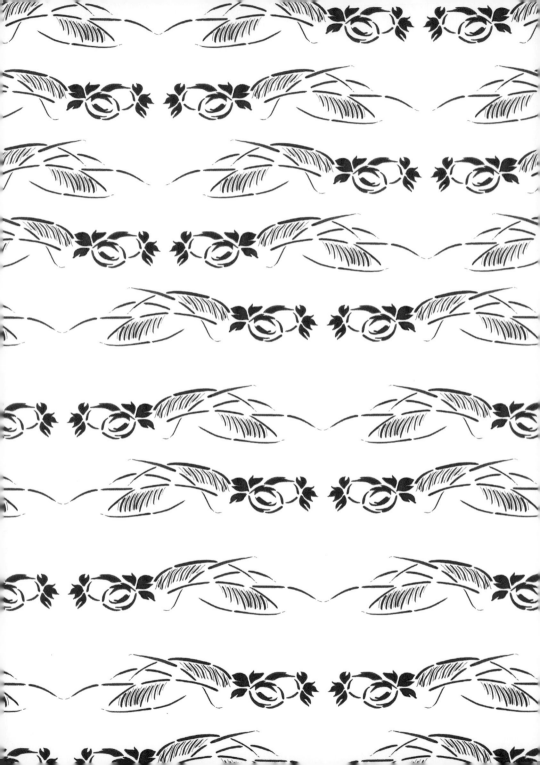

# THE JAPANESE DIET FOR CLEAR SKIN

I typically eat more when I spend time in Kyoto than I do at home, in part because dishes are so delicious and presented as beautifully as gifts. I've found that when I follow a traditional Japanese diet, my brain feels sharper and my skin looks brighter. I'm more focused and energetic, too. And my clothes certainly fit better on my body.

Most Japanese women customarily eat clean food and rely on a trinity of superfoods—green tea, rice, and seaweed—as dietary staples. Incidentally, Japan has the longest life expectancy among developed countries. Japanese women, in particular, have a life expectancy of eighty-seven years (compared to eighty-one for American women). Scientists credit their longevity to genetics but also, importantly, to lifestyle and diet.

On the pages that follow, I've shared two of my favorite simple recipes that incorporate these anti-aging superfoods.

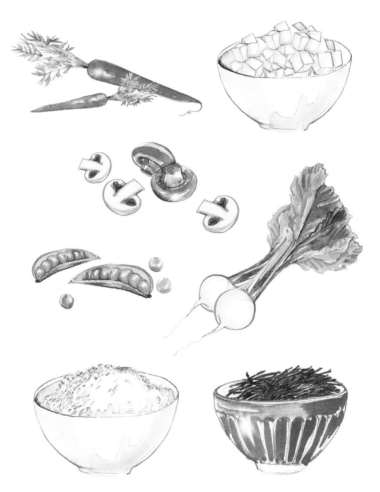

## CHIRASHI-STYLE OR "SCATTERED" SUSHI WITH GREEN TEA RICE

——

*Makes 5 servings*

I adore this recipe because you get two superfoods in one dish—and now you have a fantastic reason to clean out your refrigerator. (My daughter loves to rummage through our fresh veggie drawer and hand me ingredients.) The green tea rice makes a beautiful and flavorful base for whatever you sprinkle on top.

> *1 tablespoon green tea leaves*
> *3 cups uncooked Japanese short-grain white rice*
> *Anything in your fridge (eggs, mushrooms, carrots, snow peas, green beans, baby corn, tofu)*
> *Pinch of salt, to taste*

1. Mix the green tea leaves with the dry rice in a bowl and then cook the rice as usual. The green tea will soften on the stove and add flavor.

2. While the rice is cooking, prepare your add-in items as needed. Scramble eggs over heat and sauté vegetables like mushrooms, julienned carrots, and snow peas.

3. Once the rice is cooked, let it cool for about 10 minutes and then mix in the other ingredients. For a crunchier version, add vegetables raw and let the heated rice cook them slightly.

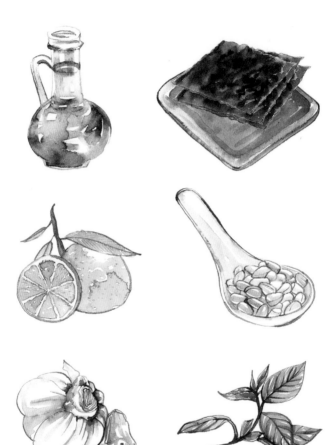

## SEAWEED PESTO

———

*Makes about 2 cups*

Reimagine traditional Italian pesto as a savory Japanese topping with this easy-to-prepare recipe. I sometimes add it to my chirashi sushi so I manage to enjoy three superfoods at once.

*5 sheets roasted seaweed (such as wakame), torn*
*½ cup pine nuts*
*½ cup olive oil*
*2 cups mixed greens (parsley, spinach, or basil)*
*2 garlic cloves*
*2 tablespoons lemon juice*

1.  In a food processor, combine the seaweed, pine nuts, and olive oil. Pulse until blended and then add the greens, garlic, and lemon juice. Pulse until well blended.

2.  Serve over rice or atop crackers, or add a dollop to poached salmon, grilled tofu, or any other protein.

# LIFE LESSONS FROM THE GEISHA

Over the years, I've spent hundreds of hours with geisha of all ages. The invaluable lessons they have taught me go far beyond skin care and even beauty, and have become philosophies I practice each and every day.

Here are the distinctly Japanese ways of thinking that I have come to value and reflect on daily, some practical and some spiritual.

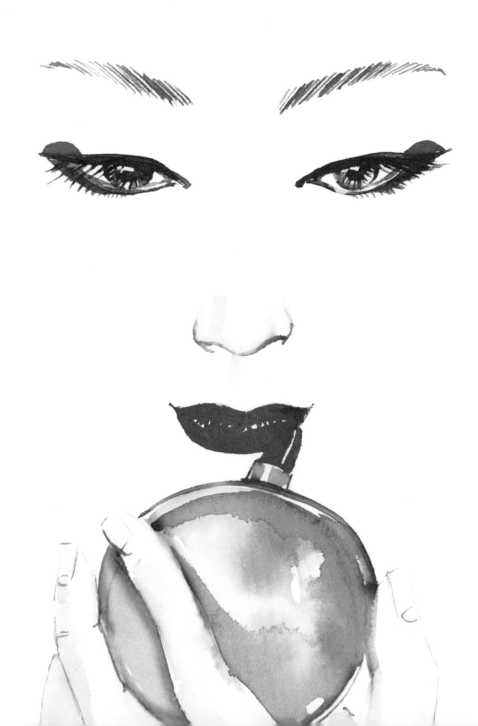

**Love your imperfections.**

Too often these days, we see skin care that promises to erase laugh lines or freckles. The phrase *wabi-sabi*, which translates to the "beauty of what is imperfect, impermanent, and incomplete," reminds us that these unique traits are part of our life stories. Laugh lines tell a story of a joyful life. Freckles are memorable and sweet.

**Embrace every birthday.**

In the modern world, it's easy to feel that your beauty fades as you age. But the geisha believe that a woman's beauty is something to be gained over time, not lost. They look up to their older "sisters" as role models and mentors. A young maiko wears ornately decorated kimono and hair-pieces, but her style becomes more simple and elegant over time. She doesn't need the accessories anymore because her beauty has become internalized.

**Love a red lip.**

A geisha's striking look isn't complete without her timeless vermilion lips. Traditionally made from a safflower extract called *beni*, this vibrant hue is precisely painted on the lips with a wet brush. You can replicate the geisha effect with dewy skin, minimal eye makeup, and a bold red lip.

**Savor each moment.**

There is a saying in Japanese: *Ichi-go, ichi-e,* or "Just this one moment, once in a lifetime." This saying reminds us of the preciousness of each interaction we have. Many physical acts we do in a day are throwaway gestures, but they can be executed with a more mindful approach. Washing your face at the end of the day can be a chore or a moment of self-care.

**Practice your posture.**

The stiff, wide obi that cinches a geisha's kimono makes it nearly impossible for her to slouch. I have also been taught to sit as close to the table as the width of my fist for perfect posture. It works.

**Toast with sake.**

If you raise a glass now and then, opt for sake for its health benefits. This delicate wine made mostly from fermented rice and water contains less sugar and impurities than Western alcohol—and no headache-causing tannins or sulfates.

**Redefine beauty.**

When you spend time with a geisha, you feel like the most important person in the room. She leans in to focus on you, and everything else falls away. In her kind eyes, you are fascinating and important. This taught me a new definition of beauty: that people remember how you made them feel. If you make someone feel cared for, you are beautiful to that person.

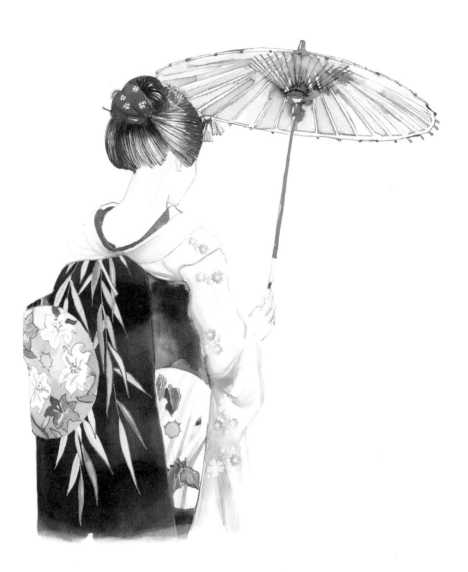

# FAREWELL

Thank you so much for joining me on this journey, which is truly just beginning for both of us. I hope you come away from this introduction to classical Japanese skin care with a new way of thinking about your skin and how to care for it.

Remember that when it comes to both your collection of products and the formulas themselves, less is always more. Enjoy the healing, meditative magic of a daily ritual, whether it's cooking breakfast, washing your face, or walking through the woods.

Perhaps most important, remember that skin care is inherently self-care. Love your beautiful skin that carries you through this world and allows you to laugh and smile.

Very few people in Japan say *sayounara* when they part because it means that you won't see each other again for a long time. I prefer a more informal good-bye, *mata aimashou.* It implies we will meet again soon. And when we do, I will want to hear *your* story. I will say, "Tell me about your skin."

*Victoria Tsai*
*Chief Treasure Hunter, Tatcha*

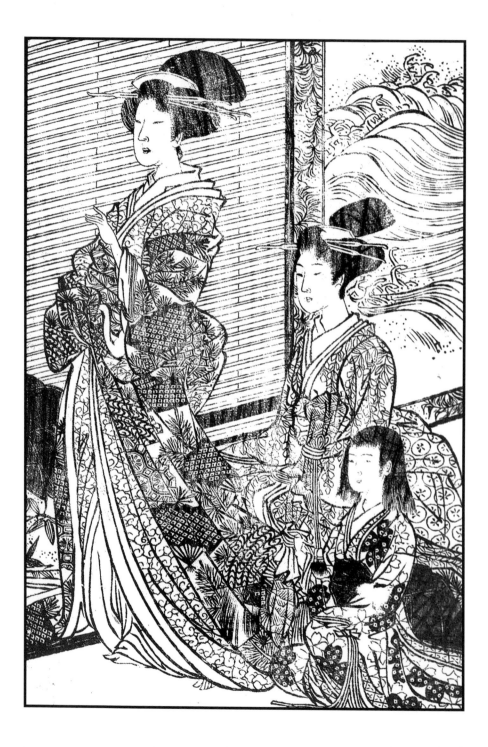

# ACKNOWLEDGMENTS

I am forever grateful to all the people who have helped me discover a more beautiful approach to both skin care and to life.

Alec Schilling, for turning this book into a reality.

Monica Corcoran Harel, for the gift of your words.

Amanda Englander, for believing that these timeless rituals could be a modern book, and the rest of the team at Clarkson Potter, for helping it become so: Ian Dingman, Cathy Hennessy, Kevin Garcia, Natasha Martin, and Stephanie Davis.

Toide-san, for being my first friend in Japan and for showing me so much kindness.

Yuko-san, for being my first guide to Japanese beauty culture and for believing in me.

President Asano and Hori-san, for sharing your beautiful world of craftsmanship and hospitality as our first partners and for introducing us to our first geisha friends.

Nami, for being the one who led us to *Miyakofūzoku kewaiden* and for dedicating your career to sharing Japanese culture with the world.

Keyin, for your beautiful eye and your tireless spirit.

The Tatcha Institute and product development team, for turning these timeless rituals into a skin care collection people can enjoy today.

Michelle Leigh, whose book *The New Beauty* was one of the first books that inspired us to dig deeper into the beautiful world she describes; and Komomo, whose book *A Geisha's Journey* captures the transformative experience of becoming a geisha in an intimate portrait. If anyone is interested in either of these topics, these are wonderful books to read.

Alea, for being my sunshine and for being so brave while I have been off treasure hunting.

None of this would be possible without the current and former geisha who have been kind enough to share their stories with us, including Oka-san, Akane-san, Toshimana-san, Marihihu-san, Mamefuji-san, Suzuka-san, Ayano-san, Satsuhi-san, Kihuno-san, Fuhunae-san, and Kyoka-san. You are inspirations to us all.

All rights reserved.
Published in the United States by Clarkson Potter/Publishers, an
imprint of the Crown Publishing Group, a division of Penguin
Random House LLC, New York.
crownpublishing.com
clarksonpotter.com

CLARKSON POTTER is a trademark and POTTER with colophon
is a registered trademark of Penguin Random House LLC.

Library of Congress Cataloging-in-Publication Data
Names: Tsai, Victoria, author.
Title: Pure skin : discover the Japanese ritual of glowing/Victoria Tsai.
Description: First edition. | New York : Clarkson Potter/Publishers, 2018.
Identifiers: LCCN 2017040113 | ISBN 9781524763336 (hardcover)
| ISBN 9781524763343 (ebook)
Subjects: LCSH: Skin--Care and hygiene--Popular works. | Beauty,
Personal--Popular works. | Self-care, Health--Popular works.
Classification: LCC RL87 .T73 2018 | DDC 646.7/26--dc23
LC record available at https://lccn.loc.gov/2017040113

ISBN 978-1-5247-6333-6
Ebook ISBN 978-1-5247-6334-3

Printed in China

Book and cover design by Ian Dingman
Illustrations by Samantha Hahn

10 9 8 7 6 5 4 3 2 1

First Edition